Dear reader:

I'm not a doctor, not a autor of anything method just want to help somebody to rid of disease. I'm living in Armenia, where, as the rest of the world, quite widespread the evils of human-the cancer. It frightens many people, but it is actually possible to prevent it. We just need to pay attention to it. The most effective method is-the removing, certain with therapy in the future. But there are many different methods that do not require surgical intervention. From a variety of methods I have chosen the method of Dr. G.Ashkar, that I consider worthy of your attention. People whose parents had cancer, are more prone to this disease. I do not have cancer /I hope that I do not have/, but because it has a genetic disposition, I am 6 months use one of the methods below-the method of Dr. G.Ashkar. I met Dr. Gashkar in Gyumri's Politechnical institute, have a talk with him, and I have use his method only to prevent a possibility of a cancer. My father died of cancer in 1992. The surgery was performed, but it was too late. In that time there were no present opportunities, there were no internet, were limited the access to big information, we didn't know a variety methods of treatment. And I'd be happy if this brochure could help even one person to rid of this disease.

I would personally like to thank the doctor G.Ashkar for his advice me and for the permission to publish this book.

M. Zadoyan

G. GREENWOOD
2020

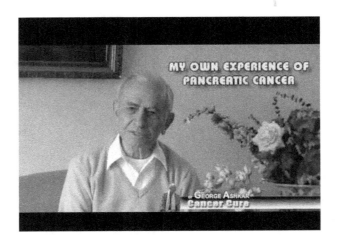

The autobiography of the GEORGE E. ASHKAR, PH.D.

On April 24, 1915 my grandfather was arrested by the Ottoman Turkish soldiers and shot to death, just for being Armenian, he was a tobacco merchant and had nothing to do with politics, my father the same day picked up all family and moved to Aleppo, Syria to avoid what happened to his father. My father could not find job in Syria, returned to Syrian-Turkish border to work in train station in Turkish side of the border. In 1916 my father married to my mother Marie Rezkalla Sayegh, in 1917 my brother Sarkis was born, in 1918 my brother Taufic was born.

All the time Turkish solders coming and asking door to door if any Armenian living there, every time my mother opens the door and telling the solders in Arabic that no Armenian living at that address.

My mother's suggestion my father decided to change our name to Arabic to avoid harassment by Turkish solders so Chilkevorkian became Ashkar, which is translation of Chil, which means red haired, to Ashkar. Misak to Elias, Vartkes to

Taufic. Changing the names to Arabic did not end the hassle. In 1919 Turkish solder knowing was my father is working decided to pick him up from train station. In the evening manager of the train station told my father to go home immediately and to not come back to work again because he got instruction to prepare all the Armenians working in train station for pick up next morning. In the next morning solders could not find my father they asked the manager were is my father, manager said that my father did not show up to work, then they asked my father's address to pick him up. Early morning they knocked my father's door as usual but this time they asked my mother by name were is my father since she realized that they know exactly were my father is living she could not foul them and asked my father to come to face the solders, Turkish solders asked my father why he did not report to work, my father said that my older brother Sarkis is sick he has to take him to doctor, luckily solders told my father O.K. take your children to doctor tomorrow morning we will come and pick you up at 9 o'clock, my father said he will report to work tomorrow, solders said to not go to work and wait at home. Next day my father was ready but it was 9;30 nobody showed up, then decided to go out to see why solders did not come, when he opened the door he saw the same two Turkish solders are shot to death in front of his door steps by advancing French solders. Because of this my father was so afraid that may they charge my father for killing Turkish soldiers. He decided to move the family to Beirut Lebanon to start new life far from Turkish border. In 1921 my third brother Antoine was born, in 1925 my sister Angel was born finally in April 23, 1931 I was born.

I attended College Saint Gregoire in Ashrafieh, Beirut, LEBANON.
On July 4th 1947 all our family, except my sister, who was

married, immigrated to Armenia in Soviet Union and settled in capital of Armenia, Yerevan. From 1947 to 1952 I attended # 44 school in Yerevan, Armenia.

In 1952 I graduated high school and the same year was admitted to physics faculty of STATE UNIVERSITY OF YEREVAN to study physics. In 1956 I was in MOSCOW STATE UNIVERSITY for six months preparing my graduation diploma in the field of cosmic rays, at physics department. In 1957 I graduated University as a nuclear physicist, specializing in cosmic rays. After graduation I was assigned to work in cosmic laboratory of the same University as senior researcher and immediately sent to city Dubna, north west of Moscow, to participate in research of structure of matter at International Research Center, using electron accelerator (of course it was for only democratic country of eastern Europe). After only two months in laboratory I was told to return home voluntarily or be fired, reason I was denied clearance to work in the research center, which considered secret. The basis for denial clearance was, unreliable foreign born citizen.
In 1959, to avoid constant denial of clearance to work in secret nuclear research laboratories, I decided to move to start research in mechanism polymerization of macromolecule, which was not considered secret field. I got position of senior researcher in VNISK, which mainly was involved in research and development of synthetic rubber, particularly in Neoprene. Here also, involuntarily, I got involved in secret research for navy. This time navy needed to cover underwater torpedoes and mines with Neoprene rubber to avoid detection by sonar, ultra sound detector, and I was the only person, who could do the work, because to do the job needed knowledge in physics, and I was the only physicist, all others were chemical engineers. Work was completed successfully; still I was denied access to see

the results of the real test, which was conducted in Baltic sea by submarine. As a promotion, I was one of the eleven participants of the patent granted for that job and received 20.00 Rubles.
In September 12, 1959 I got married to Angel Jamil Khoukass, born on January 29, 1939 in Beirut, Lebanon, father Jamil, mother Azadouhi.
In 1962 I started for my doctorate degree in Thermo-Chemical laboratory at Moscow State University after LOMONOSOV, In Moscow.
In 1965, after finishing my Doctorate degree in Chemical Physics, I got position as senior researcher at Physics Institute of Yerevan, in Armenia.
In 1965 I applied for exit visa to immigrate back to my native country, Lebanon. After being denied for many times, finally six years later on December 1970 I got exit visa.
On March 12, 1971 I immigrated back to Lebanon and on September 29 of 1971 I and my wife entered United States via J.F. Kennedy airport in New York City.
On June 21, 1977 I became American citizen.
In United States first I worked as electrician and in 1977 I was self employed and actively making research in cancer up to date.
In 1980 I find cure for cancer. In 1983 tested on woman having breast cancer spread all over the body, recuperation was 100%.

In 1985 I was arrested and convicted as a criminal for finding cure for cancer.
In 1990 I find cure for HIV-AIDS but I did not test it, since I have no formal training to deal with dangerous and contagious virus like HIV-AIDS.
In 1995 I had angioplasty surgery to place stent in artery of my heart.

In 1999 I had triple bypass heart surgery without any complication.

In 2003 I had pancreatic cancer after 5 ½ hours surgery 5 participating doctors told my wife to prepare funeral for me they had no hope to save my life. Immediately I started NIA treatment and saved my life.
On Saturday, December 1, 2007 11.00 am my wife Angel passed away in New York City, she was 68 years old, resting in Forest Lawn cemetery in Los Angeles.

TREATMENT METHOD
NEUTRAL INFECTION ABSORPTION
(NIA)

Absorption Method invented by Armenian physicist George E. Ashkar (PhD).

The idea of this (NIA) method is to artificially introduce a foreign substance into the body and let the body's immune system get in action and fight against it.

The main purpose of this method is to remove foreign particles and chemicals from the body in order to cure all chemically induced diseases.

To start the treatment we will need following materials.

  For the first time   for everyday use

1. Shaving razor
2. Plastic ring 25mm in diameter
3. or wedding ring
4. Adhesive tape
5. Fresh garlic
6. Garlic crasher
   1. Plastic Sheet
   2. Scissor (nail)
   3. Tweezers

1. Alcohol
2. Cotton ball
3. Chick peas
4. Cabbage
5. Absorbent paper
6. Adhesive tape
7. Elastic bandage
8. Gauze bandage

CREATION OF ARTIFICIAL WOUND FOR NIA TREATMENT METHOD

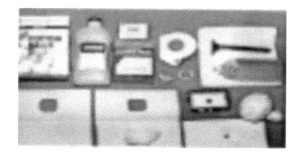

Picture-1 Material used during treatment.

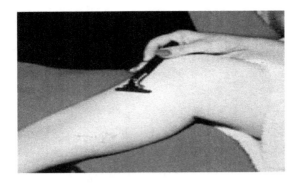

Picture-2   Shave this location to start the treatment.

We have to make artificial wound to start the NIA treatment. First we have to choose the location; the area has to be on soft muscle far from bone. Calves are the most practical place to do the wound than anywhere else on the body; it's easier to take care without help. To make it easier if you are left handed start on right calf, if you are right handed start on left calf. Shave the location approximately 6 to 8 centimeter in diameter leaving the area of the wound to be in the center. Pic.-2

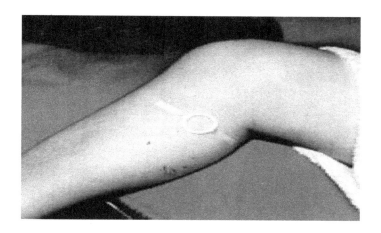

Picture-3   Fill the ring with freshly beaten garlic.

With two adhesive tapes Pic.-3 secure the plastic ring in the center of the shaved area. Plastic ring used to limit the size of the wound. Fill the ring with freshly crashed garlic evenly as high as the thickness of the ring, cover the ring with plastic sheet so that the juice of the garlic will stay inside and act to create after 6 to 8 hours a blister, sometimes you don't see blister because it happened and burst so you have to move the skin by scratching the area with sharp end of nail scissor and removing the dead skin. If you cannot find plastic ring you can use wedding ring.

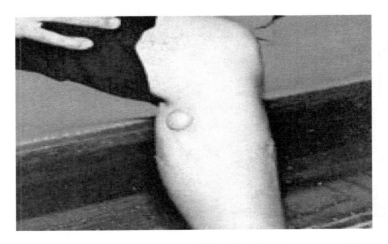

Picture-4   Blister caused by freshly beaten garlic.

After 6 to 8 hours blister will be ready Pic.-4. To avoid infection cleanup around the blister with alcohol before pealing off the skin. First make a small cut with nail scissor then peal the skin off.

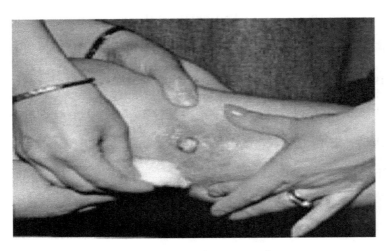

Picture-5   Chick pea in the wound.

The wound is ready. Place a chick pea in the center of the wound and cover it with a, just prepared see DVD, sandwich of cabbage and absorbing paper, napkin, so that the inside surface of the cabbage, the clean side, faces the wound and bind it with elastic bandage tight enough to not slip down when you walk, Pic.-5. For peace of mind to prevent accidental infection is better to wet dry chick pea with your saliva of the mouth for couple second then place it in the wound, this will prevent accidental infection since saliva is the best killer of bacteria, this needed because first chick pea in the wound did not yet establish flow of lymph from inside to outside the body, this flow would not give the infection chance to go inside the body. This wetting of the first chick pea is needed, you do not need to repeat every day only first one.

The body will feel the presence of the foreign substance and will fight against it by sending proper body cells to this area to neutralize it.

The chick pea will absorb the lymphatic fluid and the carcinogens and establish flow of liquid from inside out until it gets saturated and keeps the wound alive, will not let to be healed. The absorbing paper in the sandwich will absorb the excess of the fluid. In this sandwich the cabbage will keep the moisture and prevent the edge of the skin from becoming dry and sticky. This will facilitate the exchange of the chick peas.

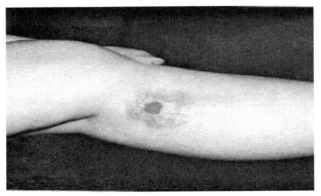

Picture-6   Wound without chick pea.

Next day, after 24 hours, open the wound Pic.-6 pull out the saturated chick pea cleanup around the wound with alcohol, insert in the wound another dry chick pea cover it with new clean sandwich of cabbage and absorbing paper, then bind with elastic bandage over the absorbing paper. Repeat the same process again every 24 hours for two days. Starting 3d day if the flow of the fluid is extensive and saturation of the chick pea comes earlier then replacement has to take place every 12 hours. The sandwich of absorbing paper and cabbage has to be replaced by a new one every time the saturated chick pea is replaced. By replacing saturated chick peas with dry one actually we are removing carcinogens and other disease causing chemicals absorbed on chick peas. This procedure has to be continued again and again until the body is cleared from impurity of foreign substances. Blood will be clean after 2 months. Depending on the length and complication of the illness it will take between 6 to 24 months to remove all trouble causing particles and chemicals from all over the body. In case if you have to take a shower, first take the shower then change and replace the chick pea, do not take shower with open wound. Wound will get infection if you leave it open more than one minute without chick pea so replace the dry one immediately without delay.

Remember never touch or treat with peroxide inside the wound, always wash your hands before replacing the chick peas. Do not need to wash chick peas or cabbage.

Time of termination can't be predicted. If no longer pus and infected blood coming out and color of the wound is normal and the main thing if you feel better then it is time to terminate the treatment. To terminate the treatment the last chick pea has to be removed and the hole kept empty, but replacement of cabbage and absorbing paper must be continued for many days until the wound is healed or treat it as a common wound Pic.-7. The sole danger in this method is the outside infection of the wound without chick peas. With chick pea inside the wound never get infection it is absolutely safe. Certain natural infection is permissible during treatment but must be very careful when wound treated without chick pea.

Since 1943 I have been testing this method to cure all types of so-called "incurable" diseases. Most of the patients were my family members, including my mother, myself and my wife, or close relatives and the diseases were arthritis related. Recuperation in all cases went up to 100% and no recurrence recorded. Since no drugs or medicines are used in this method there were no side effects, like in medical treatment, where side effects are imminent in most cases.

You have to expect following during treatment; through the wound will come out muddy liquid, pus, infected blood, all these are body's inside infection coming out of the body do not confuse with outside infection, which will never happen as long as chick peas are in the wound. Discoloration and swelling around the wound, sever pain and bad odor all these are normal do not panic all will go away as recuperation progresses, it will take time be patient. If the chick pea is not saturated it will not come out easily will stick in the wound in this case never try to pull out by using force let the chick pea stay in the wound for another day until gets saturated and pops out when you press around the wound with your fingers. Before changing the chick peas you can take a shower or swim in the sea then you change the chick peas and wet bandage, absolutely no problem...

To terminate the treatment continue the process as you were doing every day, the last chick pea has to be removed and the wound kept empty for many days until heals by itself, if there is too much infection around the wound, healing will take little bit longer until all the infection comes out completely or treat it as a common wound with an antibacterial medicine.

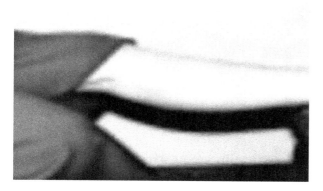

Picture7.   Closed wound after termination of treatment.

CONCLUSION

To cure cancer we have to eliminate the causation, cancer caused by carcinogens, which was accumulated in the body during years from the food we consume. Since carcinogen is not a living microorganism we cannot use drugs to eliminate them by killing, so we have to physically remove them out of the body to eliminate the causation. The only naturally treatment method, which can remove carcinogens out of the body is NEUTRAL INFECTION ABSORPTION (NIA) method, which is the only method in the world there is no alternative or substitute and it is the most perfect method and the only one. In this NIA method we are making artificial wound to access inside the body, used chick peas in the wound to keep the wound alive, and establish flaw of liquid outward and absorb carcinogens, covered with cabbage to keep the moisture around the wound to stay soft so replacement of saturated chick peas with dry ones make it easy and painless.

Presence of chick pea in the wound first keeps the wound alive and active and prevents wound from being healed and secondly causes body's immune system to get in action, pushing all carcinogens and all other particles, including cancerous cells, which do not belong to the body and could even harm, toward wound and discarding them out of the body. In two months blood is free of carcinogens and cancerous cells, but to cleanup all over the body will take at least six months and the disease will be cured 100%, in some cases it will take little bit longer if the disease is many years old or treated with radiation and chemotherapy, but definitely will be cured if it is not too late or damage is reversible.

During this treatment you can see muddy liquid, pus and infected blood coming out of the wound and smells very bad has bad odor. If too much infection accumulated around the wound you see discoloring and swelling but will go away as soon as infection gets out, that happens because too much infection is coming around the wound to get out but wound taking them out slowly sooner or later they will get out and swelling will go away. The wound itself never gets infected because of liquid flaws outward. During treatment when pus or infected blood is coming out will cause a lot of pain so you can use pain killer for relief and never any medications intended to cure cancer because radiation and chemotherapy can only cause cancer or accelerate existing cancer and never cure it. Is not recommended home remedy, vitamins, hormonal and herbal treatment also they may only slow down or stop the treatment.

WARNING. In case of diabetes take precaution, when using this method, and strictly control the sugar level to successfully heal the wound, there will be no problem.

MAGNETIC RESONANCE IMAGING

Normal cells in the body are stable, balanced and have zero polarity, as soon as healthy cell turns to cancerous everything changes. Cancerous cells are not stable, not balanced and have polarity this is the reason MRI can detect cancerous cells and only my suggested model represent them Fig.7. When we send an impulse to cells, normal cells stop, have zero relaxation time but cancerous cells, because of polarity and irregular shape, have certain long relaxation time, so MRI detecting the differences of relaxation times between normal and cancerous cells and give us the locations of these cells.

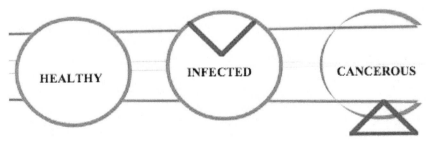

Figure-7   Magnetic Resonance Imaging

MY OWN EXPERIENCE OF PANCREATIC CANCER

I was treating people various incurable diseases, started with Rheumatoid Arthritis, Rheumatism, Breast cancer and so on, but myself never experienced any incurable diseases, which I was dreaming to have for firsthand experience. All previous were other people telling me doctor said she has breast cancer spread all over the body, after NIA treatment, again doctor said she does not have cancer in her body, all the time doctor said you have then doctor said you don't have I could not prove myself. Finally on September 23, 2003 I had pain in my upper abdomen. Next day I started vomiting and diarrhea my color was yellow my urine was black like coffee. My physician admitted me in St. Lukes Roosevelt Hospital in Manhattan, any medication to stop vomiting or diarrhea failed did not help I could not eat anything and running to toilet 6-7 times a day, lost 53 pounds in 7 days, from 195lb to 142lb. And nobody could find out what was the problem, what was going on. Finally on September 29, 2003 doctors decided to have a surgery to correct the problem. Anyway during surgery doctors found out that I had pancreatic cancer. After 5 ½ hours of surgery they cut and removed two ends of pancreas, removed and fixed tumor blocking the duck between pancreas and stomach, removed 1/3 of my cancerous stomach, removed gall bladder with stones, at the end 5 participant doctors recommended my wife to prepare a funeral for me in case. My wife told me that we do not have enough cash in the bank for funeral. I said it is very simple we do not have money for funeral I will not die so we will not need money for funeral.

After I woke up main surgeon Dr. Fadi F. Attiyeh, M.D. told me that I had pancreatic cancer. I was happy I told him very nice, he was very serious and told me chemotherapy is the only hope to save your life. I rejected immediately and asked him to discharge me from hospital to go home. Immediately I started my NIA treatment after two months my blood test to find traces of cancer were negative and still is negative. My kind of pancreatic cancer sufferer survives only 4% in the USA and 5% in the UK.

RHEUMATOID ARTHRITIS

If we compare with other diseases, we find out that Rheumatoid Arthritis has a mechanism similar to cancer the only difference is the carcinogen. This time carcinogen attacks only cartilage of the joints turning cells of cartilage to cancerous cells which get loose free and spread all over the body by metastasis, thinning the cartilage or tearing down completely. If healthy cartilage cell turned to cancerous but could not get loose free or get loose free but could not join the blood stream, then they will form soft malignant tumor around the joints and the defensive white cells will attack them in this area causing to swell and redness around the joints, which is common for Rheumatoid Arthritis. Altered cells of cartilage are not part of life sustaining organ therefore they are not causing the death because they are attacking only cartilage, which is not important life sustaining functional organ.

100% cure is available if you use "NEUTRAL INFECTION ABSORPTION" method.

COMPARISON

There are two groups of diseases caused by viral-bacterial and particle-chemical. The first group of diseases (venereal, flu, etc.) is initiated by living microorganism like viruses and bacterium. In this group diseases are transferable from one person to another by physical contact or by air. The second group of diseases (cancer, arthritis, etc.) caused by particles and chemicals (asbestos, food preservatives, etc.). These diseases are not transferable by contact or by air. If you have a single virus in your body, you never feel the symptoms of disease. Using cell's internal duplication mechanism, virus duplicates itself and accumulates in the body, you do not feel the disease, but when reaches certain "critical" amount of viruses you will experience full symptoms of the disease. To reach to "critical" amount of viruses could take between few minutes to few hours. The same is for microorganism, the only difference is, that microorganism is not using cell's duplication mechanism, instead using cells as a nutrient and reproducing itself. To cure this type of viral - bacterial diseases, since they are living microorganism, we can use medicine to kill or immobilize the viruses and bacterium in addition to the body's defense system.

If the diseases caused by particles and chemicals, mechanism is different, this time there are no duplication or reproduction, instead accumulation is, to reach to "critical" amount to cause the disease, which takes years, see NOTE. This kind of chemicals, which causes "incurable" diseases, comes inside the body and accumulates through the food we intake to survive. To cure this kind of particle-chemical diseases there is only one single method to take these particles and chemicals out of the body, there is no alternative this is the only way to cure these diseases, which is done successfully by using Neutral Infection - Absorption method. To cure these kind of diseases by using radiation or chemo-therapy, can only cause or accelerate existing cancer and never cure it, because radiation and chemo-therapy do not eliminate the cause of disease, carcinogens, instead kills the cancerous and also healthy cells and leave the carcinogens to start all over again, recurrence. Here is not so clear, you imagine if you have bacterial disease, how you can cure the disease if you destroy damaged cells and leave the bacteria alive to start damaging more and more cells.

A Survey of Unorthodox Cancer Treatments

Everyone has his own idea of just what a "quack" can be. To most of us it means a crackpot who peddles useless products at exorbitant prices. In recent years the term has been widened to include anyone who promotes a treatment which is not in complete accord with the policies or attitudes of organized medicine. People who are against fluoridation, no matter what their background, are classified by some as quacks; those who are convinced of the power of vitamin E are called quacks; an advocate of natural food in the diet is labeled a quack, etc. But the term, in its most damning sense, is reserved for those who would presume to treat cancer by means of anything but surgery or radiation. It might be an untrained country boy who has treated his local neighbors with a homemade remedy, or a bona tide researcher who has tested his treatment in a hundred scientific ways. If the medical fraternity frowns on the treatment, the treatment is finished. The developer and his associates are branded as quacks. Your doctor will be told it is a worthless treatment. He might run into serious professional trouble if he uses it. Actually how good is the treatment? Medical authorities say it is no good. The researchers say it is beneficial. He has list of patients who are willing to testify that they were helped, even completely cured, by the treatment. But once that first verdict has been handed down, nobody of any influence or authority will listen, or look at the evidence.

If the medical profession wants to find a cancer cure, why is it not willing to look for it wherever it might be? Are we to miss it because it originates in a small laboratory in the Southwest instead of the stainless steel and stone skyscraper of a multimillion-dollar research center? It is as though we had refused to use electricity because it was discovered by a publisher instead of a scientist, or refused to enjoy the Mona Lisa because it was painted by an inventor, instead of a full-time artist.

RECOMMENDATIONS

At least since 1900 all the researches, by professional oncologists, in the field of Cancer and Rheumatoid Arthritis was to not find cure for these diseases so they can keep the job and income for better living for ever. If they find cure they have to shut down all the research centers. Because I am physicist not a physician I was not interested to continue the research so I found cure for these illnesses.

NIA method is universal is not a medicine for specific illness therefore you do not have to know specific names of cancer illness. You do not need to know where the primary sources of cancer are or which part of the body metastasized to. Do not need to have expensive tests like MRI, CAT SCAN, PET-SCAN,

X-RAYS, SONOGRAM and others, which can only harm more. If you just know that you have Cancer or Rheumatoid Arthritis is enough to start NIA treatment, because NIA treatment cleans up all the particles and chemicals do not belong to the body and causing the illnesses. In general any illnesses are incurable by medicine this method is curing that illnesses 100%.

1. If you are healthy and you want to avoid Cancer and Rheumatoid Arthritis you better use NIA method at least for 6 months for prophylactic purposes because no matter what you do you will have Carcinogens in your body accumulated from the food you eat.

2. If already you have the illnesses do absolutely nothing do not use any medicine to cure them, only use NIA method and the recuperation will be 100% without any complications, problems and recurrence.

3. If you want healthy baby without any medical problems, before conceiving mother to be, not the father, must use NIA method at least for 6 months to clean up the blood feeding fetus. Clean blood grows healthy baby. If you cannot conceive to have a baby NIA method solves the problem after 6 months of

treatment with NIA method you can have baby, already many women suffering of infertility successfully had baby.

LIST OF DISEASES CAN BE CURED 100% BY USING NIA METHOD

CANCER: Breast, liver, spleen, lung, pancreas, stomach, intestine, colon, kidney, vulva, vagina, cervix, uterus, ovaries, leukemia, skin, bone, brain, prostate, testicles, bladder, nodes, mouth in one word all cancer diseases.

RHEUMATOID ARTHRITIS, Rheumatoid Arthritis, Rheumatism, Arthritis, Emphysema, Glaucoma, Bronchitis, Asthma, Lupus, Colitis and all Arthritic related diseases.

HIV/AIDS can be cured if you use (NIA) Neutral Infection Absorption method.

VERY IMPORTANT ADWISE FOR EVERYBODY
VACCINATION

Diseases can be cured but it is more important if prevented. To prevent diseases scientists invented vaccination. Vaccination can be used for single virus, if you want vaccinate for many viruses you have to make vaccine for each virus but still sometimes virus mutates and vaccine is not effective anymore to prevent the diseases so you have to make new vaccine for mutated virus. Preparing vaccine sometimes takes years.

In case of chemical diseases vaccine cannot be used since virus is not involved to induce chemical diseases and vaccine is prepared for viruses only. If you use NIA method and eliminate all chemical disease causing initiators you will get better than vaccine type prevention, since blood is clean from all kinds of initiators, all diseases has been cured for life except cancer, which will starts only when carcinogens reaches to critical concentration, naturally, not from previous cancer, only from new carcinogens we get from the food we consume. This way we cure following diseases for life: Rheumatoid Arthritis, Rheumatism, Arthritis, Bronchitis, Asthma, Emphysema never comes back, in addition prevent Alzheimer and Parkinson's diseases, also prevent Cancer at least for 10 to 15 years, at the end if you repeat NIA treatment again for prophylactic purpose you prevent having cancer for another 10 to 15 years.

Please do not hesitate to use NIA method for prophylactic purposes, this is the best way to prevent cancer, since cancer has no symptom sometimes when discovered could be too late, irreversible, therefore much wiser to use NIA method and be safe and healthy for life and it is free. I am telling that this NIA method cures "incurable" diseases 100% but cannot bring back from the funeral home therefore use it for prophylactic purposes and be safe.

You have one life to live do not count on second one.

Ladies please give us healthy babies use NIA method at least for 6 months then conceive to have trouble free healthy baby.

REGULAR CHECKUP

A regular medical checkup is a totally unnecessarily waste of time for both patient and the physician, the time could be used for more important help of already sick people who need immediate help. No one physician can say when and what kind of illness you are going to have unless it happens. If regular checkups could help to prevent an illness from occurring, first the physician himself would not get any disease and would die by natural death, which never has happened and never will happen. When you go for checkup you have to tell the doctor what kind of complain you have, not the doctor.

Suppose during a checkup, by a magic physician found out that tomorrow you are going to have Rheumatoid Arthritis. He couldn't stop it from occurring or prevent it in any ways, and if it happened, the physician has no cure for it. Then where is the importance of a checkup to prevent illness from occurring. If you have early detected breast cancer what oncologist will do? Mastectomy, which is not a cure and oncologist, has no means to eliminate carcinogens in order to cure the disease, only NIA method can do it. No one can convince me that regular checkups do save unconfirmed illnesses and no one can provide proof that illness would not occur if they had regular checkups.

There are thousands of cases where patients were rated 100% healthy by family doctors who later had heart attack and died, or had other "incurable" diseases for which physicians have neither explanation nor cure.

The best thing is to be healthy and prevent many diseases from occurring by just keeping calm to not produce promoters so carcinogen, which always you have it in your body, cannot use it to turn healthy cells to cancerous. Still, the use of NIA method, for prophylactic purpose, would be the only and the best way to avoid all the "incurable" diseases from occurring and keeping your health in the best disease-proof shape, except for inevitable, natural virus infections against which the body's defense system will take prompt action.

This method is also useful for a struggle against the AIDS.

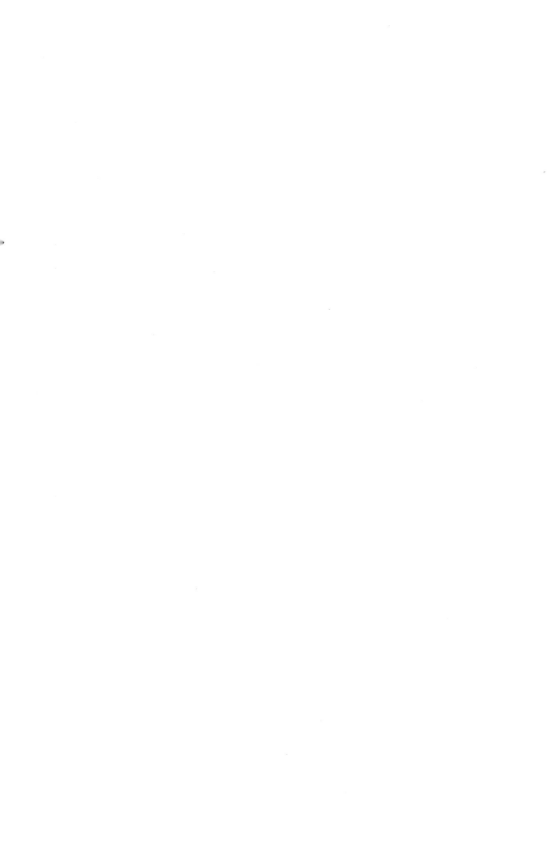

CPSIA information can be obtained
at www.ICGtesting.com
Printed in the USA
LVHW041340020920
664866LV00028B/1265